PERH

IT'S AN
ALLERGY

PERHAPS IT'S AN ALLERGY

by

ELLEN ROTHERA

W. Foulsham & Co. Ltd.
London • New York • Toronto • Cape Town • Sydney

I dedicate this book to the following committee members of the Food and Chemical Allergy Association with my grateful thanks for their most valued and loyal support over the years: Betty Hall, Betty Rogers, Margaret Shaw, Marion Tupper, and Nora and Douglas White; also to Pat Berney who would have been one if she could, and whose unfailing courage is an inspiration to us all.

W. Foulsham & Company Limited
Yeovil Road, Slough, Berkshire, SL1 4JH

ISBN 0-572-01459-7

Printed in Great Britain by St Edmundsbury Press Limited, Bury St Edmunds, Suffolk

CONTENTS

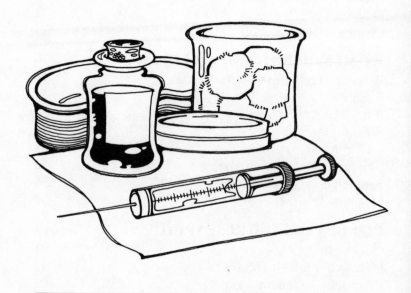

ACKNOWLEDGEMENTS

My husband David for his practical help and encourage-ment with my book and his constant moral support when I was ill. My daughter, Sally, for her efforts in producing the photograph for the cover. Doctors Richard Mackar-ness, Len McEwen and Ellen Grant for their advice. Doctor Andrew Cant and his publishers for allowing me to reproduce his *Weaning Advice*.

The Association for the Promotion of Preconceptual Care, The London Food Commission, The Food Additive Campaign Team, The National Pure Water Association, The Child Poverty Action Group, The Southern Water Authority, and Boots the Chemist, for their help with information.

Nora and Douglas White for their most valuable sug-gestions, Joan Smith for typing the manuscript with such willing enthusiasm, and John Button, my friendly, helpful and long-suffering editor.

All the people who have allowed their addresses to be included, and all the many people who have contacted me over the years, and from whom I have learned so much.

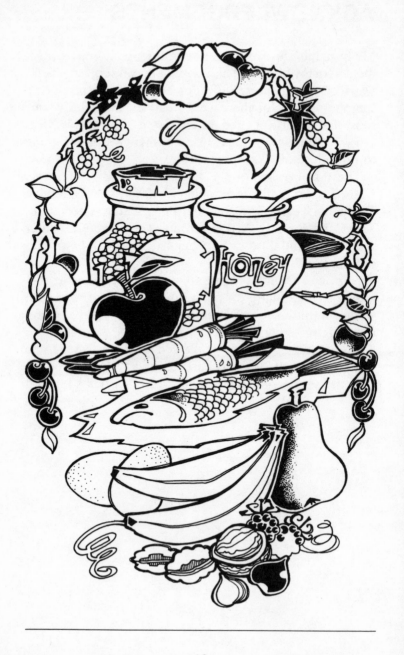

INTRODUCTION

The food and chemical allergy approach is often described as 'fringe' medicine. It is not. It is a diagnosis. As with all diagnoses, until the correct one is made the only option in conventional medicine is to suppress the symptoms with drugs.

The basic fact is that many thousands of people suffering from environmental illness are currently being misdiagnosed or are not being diagnosed at all.

Fifty years ago a relatively small number of people suffered from allergies — mainly to recognised substances such as pollens, house dust mite and moulds. These substances still cause allergic reactions today, but what so often goes unrecognised is a tide of illness caused by an ever increasing number of toxic substances encountered in our daily lives.

This realisation is not surprising since, unlike the USA where it was introduced a few years ago, the subject of food and chemical allergy is not officially taught in present day medical training. Until such time as the BMA falls in line with the thinking of other western countries on this subject, the British population suffering in this way will — in the main — have to take steps to correct its own health.

I have in my possession thousands of letters from allergic people, many of whom have met with arrogant disbelief from the medical profession. Although these sufferers would prefer to go through the orthodox channels they have, in their desperation, turned to allergy associations, often as a last resort. Some doctors may say we should not be holding ourselves up as experts and offering advice to sick people. My answer is — I quite agree! It should not be necessary.

Some people are born healthy and others have to work at it. Many abuse good health by eating poor diets which, among other things, can lead to self-induced food sensitivities. It is a tragic fact that some children are brought up on diets consisting mainly of tea, fizzy drinks and pre-packed monosodium-glutamate-flavoured snacklets. When a diet like this is combined with living in a pollution-contaminated inner-city slum, what chance do they have? None at all.

Others succumb to media advertising and starve themselves in the mistaken belief that they will look more attractive that way, thereby depriving themselves of essential nutrients. They may also develop self-induced sensitivities.

Still others eat an excessive amount of one particular food, then are ill and wonder why. Tea and coffee rank high in this form of self-poisoning; over-consumption may be due to addiction, boredom, habit or depression. If the problem can be recognised for what it is, kicking the habit is essential if good health is to be regained.

The diets that some people choose are nothing short of appalling, often consisting almost entirely of processed foods laden with chemical additives. Changing to a well-balanced diet will almost always reverse the situation and lead to an improvement in health. A good basis for any diet is water, meat, fish, pulses, fresh fruit and fresh vegetables. Given a balanced diet with these ingredients most human bodies function well.

I write this book not only for people who fall into the above categories, but also for those who, through no fault of their own, have become ill and are looking for a cause rather than simply a drug to suppress the symptoms. For anyone who suffers from an allergic reaction, I sincerely hope there will be an answer in this book to enable them to stabilise their condition.

It is essential that anyone who has any doubts or problems should consult their own doctor, a general medical practitioner, or a medically qualified clinical ecologist. As far as the latter is concerned, check what the fees might be *prior* to making an appointment.

More doctors are now becoming interested in the subject of clinical ecology. Clinical ecology is the study of the ability of the human being to adapt to the environment. There has been, for the past few years, an association for doctors only called the British Society for Allergy and Environmental Medicine, and the number of members is steadily increasing.

As more and more chemicals are introduced into the environment, human capacities for adaptation are weakening. Our only hope is for the medical profession to recognise this fact and to persuade the government that restrictions and adjustments must be made. Until this happens it is up to you, the individual, to take measures to help yourself.

No one knows what the long term effects of chemical pollution will be, but in the short term there are some people who are unable to tolerate some of these chemicals, which act as toxins upon their body chemistry. In addition to this, certain people have allergies or intolerances to so-called 'pure' foods. The most susceptible are the young, the old, and those who, as a result of the genes they have inherited, are known as allergic.

These are basic facts. Some people choose not to believe them. 'If I can eat an egg without ill effect then so can you,' is their line of reasoning. Unfortunately this is not necessarily so. Alternatively they may feel it becomes them to display a little 'healthy' scepticism.

I must confess at this point that I used to be very sceptical about the things to which *other people* claimed to be allergic. When my husband and I were first married he told me that flowers, particularly chrysanthemums, gave him hayfever, which I thought highly unlikely. So I decided I would hide a vase of chrysanthemums behind a bookcase in the sitting room. Soon after we settled down that evening he began to sneeze, gradually at first, but building up to a fine crescendo. He just could not understand it and kept saying 'but there are no flowers in here' in a bewildered sort of way. He may have had an uncomfortable evening but he proved his point!

So to all determined and dedicated sceptics, let me ask you this: is *Homo sapiens* as a species so infallible that although other forms of life may become extinct in the process of evolution, human beings can survive *any* change to the environment without ill effect?

A Word To Relatives

If you live with an allergy sufferer, whether child or adult, please read this book to give yourself a greater understanding of the patient's condition. Allergic reactions are due to a chemical imbalance which has occurred through no fault of the victim. It may manifest itself in physical or emotional symptoms and, in many cases, both. It is a very distressing illness, still little understood by the majority of people. It may be distressing for you, the onlooker, but it is even worse for the person involved.

It is possible, with time and patience, to discover and eliminate or avoid most allergens most of the time for most people, and a reasonable to good improvement in health can be anticipated. This requires considerable will-power on the part of the sufferer, and there will be inevitable set-backs from time to time. The very best aid to recovery is the support, understanding and caring of partner, parent and friends.

WHAT IS ALLERGY?

Environmental Illness or Allergy?

Environmental illness is now the number one cause of illness in the so-called civilised western world. The term 'environmental illness' is used to described all symptoms suffered as a result of exposure to something in the environment. It can be caused by an individual sensitivity — which may be an allergy — or by a substance which is toxic to everyone.

As far as allergic reactions are concerned, these can be produced by any of the following:

— Something you eat or drink (this includes medicines, the vast majority of which contain artificial colourings).

— Something you inhale (this can be natural substances such as pollens, or artificial substances such as petrol fumes).

— Something which comes into contact with your body (such as cosmetics, clothing, bedding).

— Something which is injected (such as medical injections, bee stings).

The most common form of sensitivity is a gradual build-up of symptoms resulting from regular exposure to an allergen. Where food and drink are concerned, an addictive factor is also sometimes involved.

Not all food sensitivities are caused by allergic reactions. These can also result from:

— The toxic content of the food (such as caffeine in coffee, tea or chocolate).

— The deficiency of an enzyme, which means that someone cannot digest the food properly (e.g. lactase deficiency leading to the inability to digest food containing lactose, such as cows' milk).

— Certain foods which contain a chemical which triggers off a reaction in some people (such as strawberries or shellfish).

It can be seen that the word 'allergy' relates to a specific form of adverse reaction, whereas 'intolerance' and 'sensitivity' are generic terms incorporating these three additional forms of reaction as well as true allergy.

Some doctors get rather upset if the word 'allergy' is used incorrectly, when 'intolerance' or 'sensitivity' would have been more appropriate. So, prospective patient, be warned! 'Allergy' is an emotive word! If in doubt, use one of the other two.

From the point of view of the sufferer, the need to eliminate the offending food and the means of doing so remain the same.

Anyone can develop this condition at any age. It is basically a stress disease, and can be induced or aggravated by any of the following:

— Imbalance of hormones (hence the prevalence of women sufferers, with their complicated hormone-controlled menstrual cycle).

— Infection.

— Prolonged or severe environmental stress.

— Shock.

— Nutritional inadequacy of minerals and vitamins.

— Repeated doses of antibiotics or other drugs.

— Exposure to chemicals.

In other words, a person who is in a generally low state for whatever reason is more susceptible than she or he otherwise would be. Very stressful situations, such as bereavements, can put a less-sensitive person into the category of being 'a sensitive person' for a period of time — maybe months or even years. Coming to terms with the stress will be as important in the recovery as discovering the allergens.

True allergy is a condition of the immune system which over-reacts, causing antibodies to form in the blood stream which attack the body whenever it comes into contact with the allergen. Hormones are the first line of defence against allergies, and become unbalanced in their efforts to fight the supposed foreign body. The adrenal glands produce cortisone which, if it is needed continually to counteract the stress of an allergic reaction, can become depleted. In extreme cases adrenal exhaustion may occur.

Why is Allergy on the Increase?

In 1976 Dr Richard Mackarness, a psychiatrist at Basingstoke Hospital, wrote the first book for the lay public on the subject of food and chemical allergy. Some doctors also read it, and were interested enough to visit Dr Mackerness and sit in on his clinics. Those who did so found that, when put into practice, his methods really did achieve the desired results.

I quote from the last paragraph in his book *Not All In The Mind*: 'Sooner or later, government action will have to be taken to stop the steadily accelerating drift into a harmful, chemical environment. If something effective is not done now to prevent the adaptive breakdown already afflicting more and more people in the West, we shall reach the point of no return and extinction of our complex, contaminated, improvident society will be inevitable.'

Have we taken heed of what he said? Very little has been done at an official level. But there are now many associations and bodies of people who feel strongly on the subject. There is official talk of restricting some chemicals, but others keep cropping up in the meantime. Due to a discerning public, pressure has been put on manufacturers to produce artificial-additive-free pre-packed foods, and organic fruit and vegetables are being sold in some shops. At one time nearly all ice cream contained tartrazine, but when the first tartrazine-free ice cream was sold at our local freezer shop the manager told me he could not get enough of it!

Our Association hears from very many mothers of babies and young children with genuine worries about distressing symptoms for which no answer has been found. These almost invariably turn out to be food related.

I believe that sensitivity is on the increase because, like so many things in life, it works in a vicious circle. Today's mothers have been brought up in a more polluted atmosphere than those of previous generations. They have been fed on at least some highly-processed foods with chemical additives which were not marketed a generation ago.

Thus, when they become pregnant, the foetus is nurtured in a body in which the blood stream is already contaminated with a whole variety of 'nasties', which in turn enter the baby's blood stream. Unlike the mother (since she, being physically more mature, can probably withstand what has for her been a *gradual* invasion of foreign matter), the baby faces this chemical threat from the moment of conception. The baby's immature immune and digestive systems are vulnerable to being sensitised to a host of potential allergens.

Not only that: when the baby is born, if it is bottle fed, it will have to withstand an onslaught of baby milk prepared from cows' milk which is likely to contain traces of antibiotics and hormones.

It is now estimated by some doctors working in this field that as much as 80% of the population is now suffering from intolerance of one form or another. I believe that we are evolving too fast for our own good.

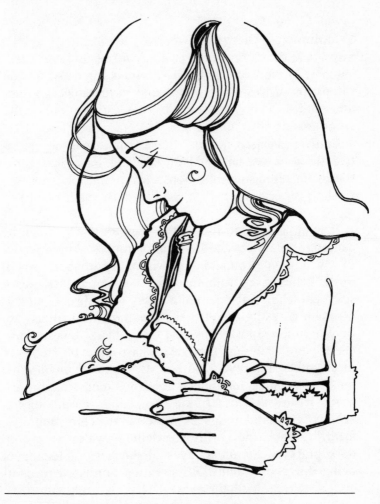

SYMPTOMS OF ALLERGY

Symptoms of Allergy

Symptoms of allergy come in many forms and can affect any part of the body. Allergic reactions can cause a wide variety of distressing physical and psychological symptoms and, in many cases, both. They can also mimic the symptoms of other illnesses.

Many clinical ecologists believe that certain degenerative diseases are allergy-induced, and have had some success in stabilising conditions such as multiple sclerosis, Crohn's disease, ulcerative colitis and rheumatoid arthritis.

It is impossible to list all the symptoms which can be caused by allergic reactions or intolerances. Among those of which people complain are: visual disturbances, weeping or itching eyes, running nose, sneezing, catarrh, sinusitis, earache, ringing in the ears, sore throat, cough, hoarseness, asthma and other breathing difficulties, abnormal pulse rate, abnormal heart-beat, palpitations, chest pains, nausea, faintness, diarrhoea, bloated stomach, other digestive disturbances, cramps, convulsions, pins and needles, numbness, abnormal menstruation, eczema, rashes and other skin complaints, mouth ulcers, aching or painful joints or muscles, twitching muscles, arthritis, backache, pruritis, swelling, water retention, dark puffy circles under eyes, drowsiness, a feeling of being drugged, exhaustion, sweating unrelated to exercise, shivering, feeling very cold, shaking, frequent urination or bedwetting, vaginal discharge, lack of libido, mental confusion, irritability, aggressiveness, depression, crying, nightmares, insomnia, hyperactivity, inability to concentrate, forgetfulness, nervousness, anxiety, lack of confidence, fears, clumsiness, food addictions, raised blood pressure, obesity, migraine, headaches, epilepsy and agoraphobia.

It is perhaps difficult for people unacquainted with environmental illness to accept that all the above can be symptomatic of allergic disease. The reason the list is so long is because people can react in so many different ways. Anyone suffering from a combination of random symptoms which do not fit a clear alternative diagnosis should always be considered as likely candidates.

At the same time, all the aforementioned symptoms can be indicative of other conditions, and everyone should be fully medically checked to ascertain that they are not suffering from something other than allergy.

Arthritis (Rheumatoid and Osteo)

I could write about any of the above symptoms, but I choose arthritis because so many people are suffering from it. Arthritis costs £1.5 billion a year in social security benefits, prescriptions and hospital services. There are two hundred research projects going on at universities and hospitals all over the country.

Everyone is looking for a cure. Why? Why do people always look for cures and not for causes? Sometimes arthritis is a by-product of another illness, such as German measles. If this is the case it will clear up by itself. If joints are damaged by injury or accident, arthritis can set in, possibly in later years. When this happens the clock cannot be turned back and the injury undone, so it is reasonable to try every possible 'cure' to relieve those distressing symptoms. But in the majority of cases, arthritis is the body's reaction to something 'toxic' which it is being bombarded with on a regular basis. If I were to

21

drink a glass of milk today, I should have two arthritic hips tomorrow. So I don't drink milk. It's as simple as that. Milk is only one possibility, albeit a common one.

In general, foods and drinks are more likely to be implicated in arthritis than inhalant allergens. If you are prepared to try out an elimination diet, you should be able to work out what is your particular poison. Listen to your body — it is trying to tell you something.

Post Viral Syndrome

Viral infections of all sorts including myalgic encephalo-myelitis and glandular fever can leave a weakened immune system in their wake, causing symptoms such as overwhelming fatigue, lack of concentration, depression, and many others. When symptoms are severe enough to warrant a diagnosis, this is known as Post Viral Syndrome. Allergic reactions can then occur to substances which were previously tolerated. In these circumstances it is worth trying to find out those things to which you have become sensitive, and avoiding them.

Office Building Syndrome

This form of illness, which can hit people who work in offices, is now recognised, but the reason for it is not commonly known. It is caused, in the main, by the use of air conditioners.

These circulate microorganisms, some of which can cause viruses. They also harbour mould, especially during the winter months, which will also be circulated, and to which some people will be allergic. They are run by gas or motor oil and, again, when this gets into the atmosphere some people will react to it. The type of air conditioners which bring in air from outside will also bring in pollens — another known source of allergen. A few days away from the office, perhaps over a holiday period, will clarify whether or not this is your particular problem.

Candida Albicans

Candida albicans (Candidiasis), or thrush as it is usually known, is a condition to which allergy sufferers are prone. Doctors often use Nystatin to combat it, and most people will respond to such treatment. Some people, however, will react adversely to it, and will have to be desensitised before it can be given without ill effect. There are others who do not respond to this treatment and for whom other remedies must be tried. Biotin, one of the B vitamins, (in conjunction with the B complex vitamins and digestive enzymes) has been found to be helpful in clearing up the symptoms of thrush.

Psychological Illness

People who use a disparaging tone when referring to psychological illness must be blessed with a poor imagination. It can happen to anyone. It may be caused by circumstances being too much for someone to bear, or a chemical imbalance, or very often a combination of both. There may also be a hereditary predisposition. Whatever the reason, the individual cannot be blamed, they are certainly not ill from choice. There, but for the grace of God, go the rest of us.

Whilst giving relief to the symptoms is essential, it is important to try to discover the basic cause. Most NHS doctors do not have time to do this, which is the reason why people so often turn to alternative therapies.

There is a great deal of misunderstanding about the psychological aspects of allergic illness. People often say that 'excitement' or 'anxiety' can bring on an attack of, say, asthma. What actually happens, I believe, is either that the emotional experience of anxiety (or excitement) lowers the allergy tolerance level so that the person will be particularly susceptible when coming into contact with an allergen, or the person is already suffering from an underlying allergy and it only needs a trigger (emotional or otherwise) to act as the 'last straw'.

At the same time, psychological symptoms can be — and frequently are — a manifestation of allergic reaction. When you think of the associated swelling of millions of brain cells, this is hardly surprising.

I believe that there are many people suffering from mental illness, or who are violent, maladjusted, or just plain bewildered, who are no more than undiagnosed food or chemically sensitive people.

We had one woman come to our meetings whose eighteen-year-old daughter was diagnosed as suffering from schizophrenia. The mother had observed over a period of time that her daughter behaved in an uncontrollable (and sometimes violent) manner after consuming either tea or Coca-Cola. As long as she could persuade her to refrain from drinking either of these, the girl behaved normally. However, from time to time, she succumbed and on these occasions had to be taken into a mental hospital. Time and again this courageous mother tried approaching the different doctors involved, telling them what she had observed, but to no avail. For all I know she is trying still.

Then there was the tragic case of the young man who was exceptionally sensitive to sugar. One day the temptation overcame him and he ate several chocolate bars. The severe depression caused by his reaction to sugar caused such overwhelming despair that he took his own life. This tragedy was brought to my notice since he lived in the same area as me; I hope his mother will forgive me for including it in this book.

I was faced with an awful dilemma soon after we started our Association, and I intend never to allow myself to be put in this situation again. A woman came to one of our meetings having discharged herself from a local hospital for mentally ill patients. She told me she had suffered for some time from severe depression, and showed me her scarred wrists. She said she was now almost convinced that food was the cause of her problems and she suspected wheat. The hospital was not interested in her theory and served her wheat with almost every meal — hence the reason for her discharging herself. She told me she was separated from her husband and could not afford to visit a clinical ecologist. Would I help her? Reluctantly, and with great misgivings, I agreed. I explained that withdrawal symptoms might be severe, but she felt it was essential to try an elimination diet in order to discover the cause of her reactions. She wanted to start at once. She rang me daily for the next few days in deep distress, threatening to take her life, and somehow I managed to talk her through it. To my enormous relief she cleared by the fifth day. Later she proved that the culprit was wheat. I do not know whether she slept at nights — I know I didn't. The last I saw of her was about a year later, when she called on me with her boyfriend. She had increased her weight from six to nine stone, looked very glamorous, and obviously had a very happy relationship with her new man.

I strongly believe, after that experience, that no one suffering from severe depression should attempt an elimination diet except under medical supervision. In practice, however, it may be almost impossible for someone to find a doctor who is willing to supervise this, unless he or she can afford the fees of a clinical ecologist. Many doctors do not believe that diet plays any part in psychological or physical illness, and this undoubtedly prevents many patients asking for help.

I have no doubt that there are many other reasons for mental illness, but sensitivity to food and chemicals must be one of the main ones.

I will include at some length the experiences of one lady who suffered this way as a result of allergic reactions, who has kindly allowed me to include them in this book. I asked her permission to do so because depression, aggression and confusion are classic psychological symptoms of allergic illness.

Depression: 'In my experience depression is always accompanied by debility, which may range from a feeling of exhaustion to a state of near unconsciousness. The combination of depression and debility is a state of total joylessness and an inability to fulfill one's obligations, combined with a terrifying feeling of the complete negation of one's personality. I found that cheer, humour and the ability to give of oneself were non-existent, and performing even minor duties required an extreme act of will. Left alone, I would sit and stare at one spot for hours on end, since everything else seemed quite pointless. I was overcome by a feeling of total annihilation, hypersensitive to all that was going on around me but quite unable to communicate.'

Aggression: 'For me, the state of aggression was always accompanied by an involuntary tightening of the stomach muscles. This condition ranged from feeling rather disagreeable to feeling quite violent. There is an all-consuming feeling of "what the hell," and I found it better to be on my own whenever possible. Any frustration, however minor, caused a rush of what I assume to be adrenalin pulsating through my veins. I could feel this happening. For those who can express themselves verbally, this relieves the terrible tension. I put my family through hell. It was only with the greatest act of will power that I did not attack them physically.'

Confusion: 'In this condition, my mind was unable to assimilate all but the simplest of facts. To follow my basic routine out of sheer force of habit was as much as I could achieve. I found myself nodding and smiling during conversations without having the slightest idea of what people were talking about. My mind was turned inward. I saw without perceiving, people's names became confused, and I could remember only those people who were familiar to me. In this state I was unable to express myself

26

because I could not remember the words I knew I wanted.'

I challenge any doctor reading this book who has patients suffering from mental illness to give them a chance of recovery by using the food and chemical allergy approach. Can he or she in all conscience deny these lost souls a final opportunity before being condemned for ever to the fear, bewilderment and total despair of the terrifying twilight world of the mentally ill?

Violence

I am not surprised at the horrific heights of criminal violence we have reached in this country. I believe the main contributors to this situation are:

Lack of Discipline: Since the Victorian days of strict discipline, the pendulum has swung right over to the other extreme. Some parents do not even teach their children the difference between right and wrong. They are allowed to be destructive or attack other children without being reprimanded. This is called being 'progressive' and was very much in vogue when I was bringing up my youngest child.

Influence of Television: More time is spent by children and adults watching TV than any other single pastime. When you consider the abundance of films portraying killing, sadism and oppressive promiscuity, together with the fact that some immature people are receptive to trying out these new ideas, it is not surprising that some actually put into practice what they have seen.

Environmental Toxins: If people take too much alcohol, or indulge in drug-taking or inhale solvents, they must know that they are courting danger. These are all major contributors to violent behaviour. But people *do have a choice*. What most people do not know is that some foods (such as sugar), chemicals in foods (particularly artificial colourings), or chemical inhalants are going to cause certain susceptible people to become violent. In the majority of cases when this happens they will not know why, and will therefore not be in a position to prevent it happening again. Our bodies have become so saturated with the toxins in our environment that even if this situation were to be accepted and dealt with now, it would probably be many years before any improvement would be noticed.

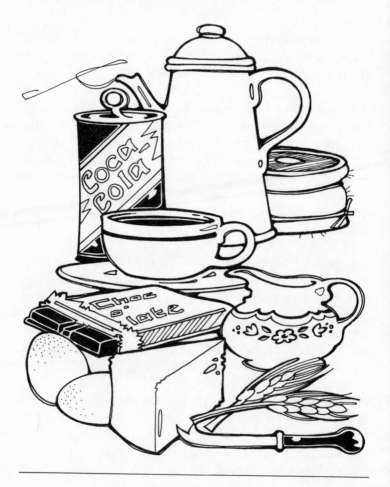

ALLERGENS

FOODS

Anybody can be allergic to anything. No two people are the same, although two closely related sensitive people can have overlapping allergens. However, there are certain foods and drinks which have higher allergenic properties than others, and are therefore more likely to cause problems. Among these are coffee, tea, chocolate, Coca-Cola, milk and milk products, cheese, eggs, pork, fish, potatoes, peas and beans, cereals (particularly wheat and corn), sugar, soya, yeast, and citrus fruits and citric acid.

Coffee, Tea, Chocolate and Coca-Cola

Coffee, tea, chocolate and Coca-Cola all contain caffeine. Caffeine is a known stimulant, and anyone who needs to take sleeping pills should consider whether this might not be part of their problem. It is not sufficient to say 'I do not drink coffee before I go to bed' because the effect can be longer lasting than that. I suggest that all insomniacs try giving up these drinks for a week to see if this produces the desired results.

Apart from the caffeine content, coffee, tea, chocolate and Coca-Cola are high in allergenic properties anyway, added to which chocolate contains tyramine. In powdered coffee, two additional potential risks can be responsible for causing an adverse reaction — the chemical processes it has gone through to become 'instant', and the chemicals added to it to present and preserve it in its powdered form. Studies have been done which show that heavy coffee drinkers raise the level of cholesterol in their blood, thereby making them more prone to heart attacks and strokes.

Everyone, including non-allergic people, has a caffeine consumption limit, and high doses can produce symptoms of the central nervous system. Anyone suffering from 'nerves', anxiety, shakiness or apparent heart symptoms might do well to consider how much caffeine they consume. Even the smallest amount can affect some susceptible people. Caffeine is also to be found in certain medications; it is added to pep you into feeling better when you are not, and thereby seducing you into buying the same medication again.

Cows' Milk

Cows' milk, taken in moderation, is an excellent food for those who can take it. Unfortunately, some people cannot. It is one of the main causes of allergic illness in humans — we being the only species who consume the milk of another mammal.

Cows' milk is known, among other things, to be associated with some cases of infantile eczema, and a range of intestinal problems. Ulcerative colitis, for example, has often been treated with a bland milky diet when actually the very cause can be an inability to tolerate cows' milk! The allergy to cows' milk can be due to the casein (the protein in milk) or to the whey (the opaque liquid left after the casein and fat have been removed). Some of the allergenic properties of milk are destroyed when it is heated to a high enough temperature. For this reason, some milk-allergic people may be able to tolerate evaporated milk.

At present the dairy industry in Britain, with government support, is considering increasing milk yields with the use of the hormone Somatotrophin. The EEC already

INDEX